ONE OUT OF EIGHT

NO GENES REQUIRED

JOYCE MCCHESNEY-KAYE

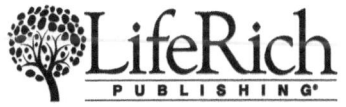

LifeRich Publishing is a registered trademark of
The Reader's Digest Association, Inc.

LifeRich Publishing books may be ordered through booksellers or by contacting:

LifeRich Publishing
1663 Liberty Drive
Bloomington, IN 47403
www.liferichpublishing.com
1 (888) 238-8637

Because of the dynamic nature of the Internet, any web addresses or
links contained in this book may have changed since publication and
may no longer be valid. The views expressed in this work are solely those
of the author and do not necessarily reflect the views of the publisher,
and the publisher hereby disclaims any responsibility for them.

Any people depicted in stock imagery provided by Getty Images are
models, and such images are being used for illustrative purposes only.
Certain stock imagery © Getty Images.

ISBN: 978-1-4897-1597-5 (sc)
ISBN: 978-1-4897-1596-8 (e)

Print information available on the last page.

LifeRich Publishing rev. date: 03/14/2018

I DEDICATE THIS BOOK TO TEAM, "GOT HOPE!"

Barbara
Tanya
Kriss
Cheryle
David
Linda
Martha
Nancy
John
Suzanne
Trish

PREFACE

After being diagnosed with breast cancer, I began to keep a diary. Partly in an effort to keep my sanity and partly in an effort to express my fears and frustration. I was not only blindsided by the commonality of this, but I had no idea what women were expected to endure, and I don't believe most people do.

I decided that I needed to shout from the rooftops what I learned regarding the risks. Share my crazy experiences and make my fears known. Why? Because this is a year-round topic; not just meant to be discussed during the month of October, which is designated as breast cancer awareness month. Because I've never heard anyone express their fears. Why is that? Because I'm not the only one to experience some less than ideal circumstances and frankly, women deserve better.

Friends and family have always filled our lives. They help make our world whole. We get together for Holidays, Weddings, Graduation and Birthdays. We are there for one another when parents pass. We lean on each other when children are sick or in a predicament. But when faced with breast cancer, I discovered they had no idea what to do and they had no idea what to say.

Well, maybe it's time for everyone to learn.

My breast cancer was not unique. I believed it was one of the most common diagnoses regarding breast cancer. But the hurdles and challenges I faced along the way were not at all common. It made my experience even more difficult and challenging. Friends and family didn't see this. Friends and family do not see, hear or experience what you and I experience. If they heard all the stories that I have, they would think I was telling tales, but I'm not.

So, I'm being brutally honest with my fears, thoughts, and experiences. Not because I think they are unique but because I believe they are all too common and no one speaks of them.

This book is for the friends, family members and co-workers of those who have been diagnosed with Cancer; more specifically breast cancer. Learn from my experiences, and the experiences of others I have met along the way, how you might best help. Learn what to say and what not to say. Learn what you can do to make a difference. Some of the simplest things could brighten your loved one's day.

This book is meant to help my family and friends, as well as yours, learn. This book is for them, not the newly diagnosed person.

Everyone knows or will know someone affected by a life-changing diagnosis or a life-changing experience.

As they say, until you walk in my shoes......

INTRODUCTION

Last year, I was diagnosed with Breast Cancer. I was completely and utterly blindsided by this. I had always been concerned about high blood pressure, heart disease and diabetes due to my family history. Breast Cancer was the one thing I thought I didn't have to worry about. Boy, was I wrong!

Once diagnosed, what I learned had my head spinning. According to BreastCancer.org, 1 out of 8 women will be diagnosed with breast cancer in their lifetime. Absolutely staggering! Even more staggering to me is that only 15% of the cases are genetically related. Who knew? Not me!

Why did I not know that? Why have I thought for years that breast cancer was, for the most part, genetically based? Isn't it all about the BRCA gene? Well, I didn't have the BRCA gene, but I sure had Breast Cancer.

I wanted to shout what I learned from the rooftops! But who am I? So, I began to write; in order to help me maintain my sanity.

When you are first diagnosed, everyone rallies around and tells you, "how easy it was for their friend," "it was piece of cake for my neighbor" or the one I really loved, "you're lucky, they caught it early." Easy to say for those who aren't staring that "C" word in the face.

I'm here to tell you it sucks! For me, it may have been caught early, but I never felt lucky and there was nothing easy about any of it, I'm sorry to say.

I began to wonder why I had never heard anyone speak of their cancer treatment and how they felt about being diagnosed with cancer. I know a few people who have battled this beast and yet, I've never heard them speak of it. I've never heard the stories from those "friends and neighbors."

What I did discover is that if you worry or complain or say anything other than, "No Biggy," you are acting like a three-year-old having a temper tantrum. True Story! Expressing your true feelings isn't politically correct, or something like that.

You are supposed to dutifully get on the conveyer belt and be grateful. Grateful that hardly anyone dies from breast cancer anymore. Lucky, that so much is known about breast cancer. Thankful, because it could have been so much worse. More true stories!

Whether anyone is grateful, thankful or lucky, dealing with cancer is just hard. It's a long road with twists and turns. It isn't just one surgery, one treatment or one trip to the hospital. It's a full-time job with endless side effects. Who would sign up for any of that?

Who woke up one morning and said, "no problem, I've got extra time on my hands," "I don't mind subjecting myself to radiation or having harsh chemicals run through my veins"? "Be damned my job. Who needs to pay those bills?" You are supposed to just grin and bear it. I know, what's the alternative? But why are we expected to smile through it all and never express our worries, fears, side-effects and concerns?

So, let me set the record straight. It's OKAY to be mad. It's OKAY to be angry. It's OKAY to feel you have been dealt a lousy hand. Don't let anyone tell you or make you feel otherwise. And it's OKAY for you to express your fears.

After all, it's that "C" word; cancer.

As if being diagnosed with cancer isn't hard enough already, for some reason, that group of supporters will just disappear; no cards, no flowers, no emails. I suppose they may not know what to say or do, but neither do you. I suppose they are just too busy—after all, breast cancer is quite common. It can't be that big of a deal, right? Wrong! Just ask my friend who will spend a total of 15 months receiving chemotherapy.

Others I believe think, if we don't talk about it, it isn't real. If we ignore it, it never happened.

Being diagnosed with breast cancer can be one of the loneliest and longest years of your life; it was for me.

Eventually, you will find other breast cancer survivors. There are blogs and support groups and National Organizations that are there to help. Breast cancer survivors seem to only speak amongst themselves. But, it's a club you don't want to belong to.

Other than Breast Cancer Awareness Month, when does anyone tell you that next year's mammogram could change your life? It is a life-changing diagnosis. There is no cure for cancer! There are treatments, but this ugly beast can come at you time and time again.

That's the dirty little secret about breast cancer, the bastard can keep coming at you. Just ask my other friend who had a mastectomy, and the beast returned six years later.

My story isn't just about breast cancer. It's about support, understanding, and compassion. This is true about any life-changing diagnosis and there are plenty of them out there. I'm just telling it through my eyes and my experience. But you can change the disease, and the feelings and emotions will be the same.

I'm telling my story for three reasons:

1. Understand the real risk of Breast Cancer; don't be blindsided as I was.
2. Learn how to brighten someone's day and show support to someone you love.
3. Understand what not to say to a newly diagnosed person and not stick your foot in your mouth like so many that came before you.

So, think before you speak. Don't offer false hope. Continue to be there to support your loved one, and not just in the beginning. And understand, sometimes the silver linings are very hard to find.

Make time in your busy day.

Try to walk in our shoes for just a moment.

This could be you, your wife, a friend, or even your daughter. At any given moment, this shoe could be on your foot.

Hope that you are not next year's statistic.

Because each year it is, "1 out of 8 women," period, the end! No genes required!

FAT, DUMB & HAPPY

For years, we women have dutifully gone to the gynecologist—that dreaded yearly trip that is worse than the dentist. You have your Pap smear and head home expecting that letter to come in the mail saying, "All is well, see ya next year."

Then you get a little older and a new yearly visit called the mammogram is added. This big, ugly machine is made up of desk supplies that I'm certain some man invented. You are standing on your tiptoes just waiting for this machine to pick you up off the ground, while one breast is being compressed between what looks like two desk file trays. You head home and wait to receive that letter that states, "All is well, see you next year." Some of us have received that heart-stopping letter that says, "You have dense breasts, come on back." What does that even mean? So, you call and make another appointment, and this time they have the radiologist read it on the spot and you are all set for another year. After 15 years of mammograms, I believe I have received that dense breast letter at least seven or eight times.

Then one day you again receive that heart-stopping letter that says come on back. This time it was New Year's Eve 2015. You call and make another appointment just as you have done many times before. But when appointment day arrives and you check in, something is somehow different. I'm thinking, this is a completely different waiting and changing area. First off, they reimage only one breast. Then they take an ultrasound. Instinctively you know something is wrong. That letter had no signs of urgency. That letter was like all the previous letters. Then they take you into another room and state that they saw something and a biopsy needs to be done. That was February 1, 2016.

There you sit, in that drafty hospital gown, sweating, with heaven knows what hanging out, feeling all alone, with a stranger telling you that cancer could be a distinct part of your future.

So, in a panic you call your husband, sister, or best friend right away, and, of course, your loved ones are just as blindsided as you and no one knows what to say. Your mind is running wild. The nurses at the breast care center are telling you that the chances are small, and that only about 20% of biopsies come back as breast cancer. That does offer a bit of momentary relief.

Cancer? How is this possible? There is no history of cancer, let alone breast cancer, in my family.

The clock begins to tick on the longest year of your life.

PEOPLE DON'T ALWAYS NEED ADVICE

At first, I only told my husband and my sister. After all, there was only a 20% chance of this blip being cancer. They tried to be supportive with, "It won't be cancer" and "don't worry." Seriously? I guarantee if someone mentioned cancer to you, worry would be at the top of your list! You can't help but worry.

Those much younger than me may feel that the word cancer is only slightly frightening. I was born in 1960. When Dad came home from work at the end of the day we sat around the dinner table together, and he would say to Mom, "Oh, I forgot to tell you, Mrs. Docherty has cancer." No one used the word breast in those days. Mom would respond, "I wonder which funeral home they will use?" In the 60s and 70s cancer was a death sentence. They didn't have the diagnostic technology that is available today. They didn't have the treatment that is available today. They never caught it early. It wasn't until the early 1970s that mammography became generally available, and it didn't become routine for many years. My own mother never even had a mammogram. Cancer back then never had a good ending.

Despite knowing that the technology is different and so advanced, you can't help but remember those dinner conversations. You haven't yet had the biopsy let alone been diagnosed, but the thought of cancer is heart stopping. It is now up close and way too personal.

I understand that it's people's first instinct to think positively. Friends and family rally around like a bunch of cheerleaders with, "think positive thoughts," or "you must believe your glass is half full" or "it won't happen to you." Like what I think or feel is going to change anything, particularly a medical diagnosis. I'm supposed to close my eyes and think about pink unicorns, and the biopsy won't be cancer. Oh, please, are you clairvoyant?

I suppose this is their defense mechanism. A way to protect themselves. Think happy thoughts and only good things will happen. But let's at least be realistic. You, my family or friends, just don't know which way it will all turn out. Being told "don't worry" is not realistic. You will fall that much harder and that much further when all you have been told is, "don't worry, it won't happen to you." Be very careful with the words you choose. Do not offer false hope. This is cancer after all. Only a fool wouldn't be worried.

Your mind will begin to go wild and work overtime, and the longer you must wait for the biopsy and the results, the crazier you will become. Unfortunately, I had to wait 18 days for an available biopsy date. My anxiety became worse each passing day.

I began to do some double checking with a few relatives to confirm who in my family, if anyone, had cancer, or more specifically, breast cancer. There was no history. Neither side of my immediate family had a history of breast cancer. So how is this possible? Oh, I did have a first cousin who had breast cancer 15 years ago, but she was taking hormone replacements during perimenopause. Well, that explains that. Why am I worried? My doctors had always dismissed this. And my doctors also dismissed Dad's prostate cancer, I guess because I'm a girl. I would later learn how very wrong I was.

As I waited those 18 long days and 18 long nights, I began to lose my mind. I wished my family had done some thinking for me instead of telling me not to worry. I know they were not experts at this, but neither was I. They were trying to be strong for me. They were trying to encourage me. I had put my faith and trust in my medical facility. But, there are many other facilities and centers that could have performed this biopsy, I would learn. I shouldn't have had to wait 18 days. But I wasn't thinking clearly. Instead of offering me platitudes and false hope, I wish they had thought to pick up the telephone and find another facility that could perform this biopsy much sooner.

I barely slept for 18 nights.

Then, I began to fight with myself, and I didn't even yet have a cancer diagnosis. I merely had an image with what appeared to be a dust bunny on the screen. I thought, maybe I'm worrying too much. Maybe it is like in the movies, the machine was broken. The doctors are wrong! But, what will I do if it is cancer? A million thoughts traveled through my mind. Then I realized what I had been told— only a 20% chance of cancer. Holy crap! That is not a *slight* chance! If I had a 20% chance of winning the lottery, I would play, daily! If you were told there was a 20% chance that you would be hit by a bus today, would you leave your house let alone cross a street?

Your mind will run wild with every possibility you can imagine. My manicurist, who had endured breast cancer, happened to call me during my marathon waiting period for my biopsy. I just melted like butter on a griddle and told her everything. Over the next many months, falling apart and crying would happen when least expected. I could barely speak without becoming choked up. She told me to stay off the Internet. Sound advice at this point. You do not yet have a diagnosis, so what exactly would you research? Breast cancer, I would learn, has so many twists and turns. It would have made me crazier had I not listened to her. I was out of my mind just waiting for this biopsy.

You can't get away from it either. The commercials each evening are relentless; for example, the woman taking her chemotherapy through a port in her arm with the dog wanting to go for her walk. Or the lady taking multiple medications due to metastatic breast cancer. Suddenly you hear loud and clear the radio ads in search of those harmed by XYZ type of chemotherapy, which caused permanent hair loss. And you now pass many women in the bank, grocery store, or pharmacy who are wearing beautiful scarves or hats on their heads, and it has nothing to do with religion. Or they have a military-style haircut and they are most definitely not in the military. You don't want to stare, but you never noticed this before, at least not this many women. And you wonder, will that be me?

It is everywhere! The evening news features a woman who won a game show but lost her battle with cancer before her taped episodes aired. Or the news will tell a story of yet another young lady with cancer who was a young, vibrant body-builder, but now she is in her third round of treatments and weighs barely 90 pounds. Different cancers, yes, but none of them had a positive outcome. These commercials and advertisements are endless.

How can you not be worried with this all around you?

It's that C-word. Cancer.

We don't want to hear about the fun hats or beautiful scarves that you will buy for us. We don't need your opinions or feelings We need your compassion and understanding. We need a friendly smile. We need your brain to help us navigate. We need your ears to listen. We need your shoulder to lean on and arms to hug us.

This isn't about your thoughts or your feelings. This is about us! We must endure it and live through it. You don't. Merely ask how you can help and be there to support us through it all and to the end.

And please, stop with the clichés; "you are strong and I know you can get through this" or "you're tough, you can beat this." What if we don't or what if we can't beat this? Then what? We need answers, not cheerful speculation or metaphors.

Over the next few months, I would meet and speak with women who endured breast cancer or the scare of breast cancer. Time and time again, these women confirmed to me the same fear that I had felt. They too admitted it was all overwhelming and sometimes downright terrifying. They understood my fears. It takes time to meet these women and to hear about their emotions. They too have the same fears that you do. It helps to know you are not alone. It helps to know your fears are not irrational.

Your supporters do not understand this fear unless they have been down this road, but most haven't despite the statistics. People have good intentions but cheerleading does not become them. They have the wrong handbook. Even the most cheerful and happy person will have emotions when confronted with a cancer diagnosis; who wouldn't?

Fear is a cruel beast. Think long and hard about the last time you had such worry or stress. Was it waiting for the pediatrician to call when your child had that 100 plus fever? Or maybe it was when you were waiting for AAA to arrive when your car broke down on that dark country road. Maybe it was when a parent was gravely ill. Or could it have been that large polyp that was removed during your colonoscopy and the pathology report was lost in the mail? Did these events in your life have you pulling out your hair? How many commercials did you see about the pediatrician taking too long to call back? How many radio ads did you hear about colonoscopies? And the word cancer was never personally directed at you during these trying moments in your life, was it? Now ask yourself, if someone had directed that "C" word at you, would you be patient and reasonable?

This endless wait was breaking my spirit. This endless wait was breaking my fight.

I didn't even know yet if there was anything to be concerned about, but the thought of being diagnosed with cancer wasn't just scary, it was downright terrifying. Biopsy day will come and biopsy day will go. You will hope and you will pray, but none of that will matter. God can't help you now.

I thought that was the 18 longest days of my life. I was wrong.

KEEP CALM AND FIGHT ON

Finally, biopsy day arrives. Heaven knows it was the last place I wanted to be, but I had waited 18 long, agonizing days and nights. They were mostly sleepless nights as well. I would wake up in the middle of the night in tears. But what was I worried about? There is no breast cancer in my family.

I must admit, my biopsy was not a challenge. It didn't hurt a bit and I barely knew that they were removing tissue from my breast. I only mention this because I understand that many others have a much more difficult time, and some institutions use a mechanism that makes a horrendous sound that is quite unsettling. But no matter what process they use, they all pat you on the head and send you on your way and promise to call as soon as they know anything; two to four days. My biopsy was on a Friday, so I continued to be sleepless for four more nights.

During my entire adult life, I have completed countless health forms. These forms have all sorts of little boxes and lines for you to complete your family's medical history. Please tell us about your mom, dad, brothers, sisters, grandparents, and children. I reported heart disease, stroke, and high blood pressure, time and time again. What about my uncle with diabetes? Nope! What about my cousin with cystic fibrosis? Nope! Well, how about my father's prostate cancer when he was 70? Well, not really, nope. Well, that is just not correct once you are diagnosed with breast cancer. Apparently, prostate cancer and breast cancer can be linked to the same gene. Why had my doctors not mentioned this before? That's significant. Fortunately, that gene tested normal for me. My first cousin's breast cancer was so vital to my personal history that it was good enough for the insurance company to agree to pay for a full genetic panel for me. Apparently, the first-cousin connection is quite significant after all. How did I not know this? Why have my doctors dismissed these things in the past? Why was it not important before but now it is vital information?

Tuesday afternoon, my cell phone finally rings, and you know by the caller ID that this is it. I was at work. I had continued to work and do all my usual activities just to keep busy and to keep from going MAD. All those words of encouragement and denial from my chain of supporters came crashing at my feet. THEY WERE ALL WRONG! I had breast cancer! Why did I even listen to a single word they said? I was just pushed off a cliff and I have no idea what is at the bottom. NOT YET!

I don't even remember driving home. I was devastated. Now what?

I later learned that approximately one out of eight U.S. women (about 12.5%) will develop invasive breast cancer in their lifetime (Breastcancer.org, 2017)—basically, 250,000 women in any year. Start dividing that by the number of states and counties and so on. For me, that meant five women in the town where I live will be diagnosed this year with breast cancer. I live in a small town. That may not seem like a lot, but if it were you, it would be one too many. And, some 40,000 plus women will die each year. That's significant. That means nearly 800 women from each state will die from breast cancer each year.

I live near the ocean, and each year JAWS swims by and causes "us" a bit of anxiety. Because of this, the other week I heard, on the local radio station, that according to the University of Baltimore the chances of being attacked by a shark are 1 in 3.7 million while the chances of getting hit and killed by a car are 1 in 90 and the chances of catching the flu are 1 in 63. Did you get a flu shot this year for this 1 in 63 risk? Just saying!

Today I heard a radio ad regarding autism. The ad compared the odds of winning the Grammy to the odds of children with autism. The risk is great—1 out of 110 children will be born with autism. The thought of children going through anything is sad. Those are very significant odds. But let's think back to the odds of being diagnosed with breast cancer—1 out of 8.

Absolutely staggering!

Even more staggering to me was that only 15% of the cases are genetically related (Breastcancer.org, 2017). You could have knocked me over with a feather. Why did I not know that? Where are the TV commercials with these statistics? Why have I thought for years that breast cancer was genetically based? Isn't it all about the BRCA gene?

Why has no one mentioned these statistics? I found these numbers quite easily when I finally began to look into it. One out of eight is not on any evening commercial. Did I miss the movies telling me it isn't all about genetics? I do not recall my gynecologist or primary care physician mentioning this risk. They only ask if I had my yearly mammogram. Did I neglect to read some pamphlet that they gave me? If it was on a daytime talk show, I was working! I've watched the commercials during the month of October, which is Breast Cancer Awareness Month. Did I hit mute while they were telling the world about the high-risk factors and statistics to women while they were selling those ties?

One out of eight women will be diagnosed with breast cancer in their lifetime. Only skin cancer is more prevalent at 1 out of 4. Where are the warnings that "next year's mammogram could change your life forever?" Forget the ties! Just display on the television screen, "1 out of 8 women, period, the end! No genes required!"

I, of course, went for my yearly mammogram. I did my

self-exams. It just wasn't in my family history. I thought breast cancer was the one thing I didn't have to worry about. How very wrong I was. I never once gave a thought to breast cancer. Why? Could it be hearing about Angelina Jolie and the BRCA gene made me think it was all about heredity? Well, I don't have the BRCA gene, but I had breast cancer.

After my primary care physician gave me the news, he suggested that I see a particular surgeon. He was going to contact this surgeon right away and "pave the way." They would call me the next day to set up the consult. The phone never rang.

Really? What next?

When I telephoned this surgeon's office, I was told he no longer performed lumpectomies. Needless to say, my world crashed a bit further, but I learned a valuable lesson. Don't depend on anyone. Take control, because so much is out of your control.

I took control and decided to interview multiple surgeons. My husband and I got on the phone and made appointments. We all were thinking again. With the help of my sister's neighbor thousands of miles away, we would end up at one of the best facilities with what I feel was the most wonderful surgeon. She made me feel important. She made me feel as though I mattered.

When you are diagnosed with breast cancer or any cancer for that matter, you feel time is of the essence. You want the surgery and you want it now. No one wants to walk around with cancer and say, "It will wait, no problem, no rush. I have all the time in the world to take care of this." Nonsense. You are all but ready to cut it out yourself with the steak knife in your kitchen.

Time does not seem like a friend.

It took one to two weeks to get the appointments with these surgeons, but two of the three surgeons I met with couldn't operate for another 30 days, which would be the first of April. That, too, added to my anxiety.

When I look back, I have to wonder why it took 18 days to get a biopsy. Are there that many potential cancer patients? That's a very scary thought. Why were the surgeons so booked? A multitude of lumpectomies and mastectomies? That is an even scarier thought. It will make you think. It will make you wonder. Frightening!

Not everyone has multiple facilities from which to choose, but there are alternatives out there. Some of us have several and others may have only a few or maybe even none, so help your newly diagnosed cancer patient any way that you can. But don't settle. Find the right doctor for you. And don't wait. The waiting will do more harm than you can possibly imagine.

While going down the medical rabbit hole called breast cancer, I was told by other breast cancer patients and survivors how they too eyed that steak knife in the kitchen. Why had I never heard these stories before?

It was so helpful for me to hear the stories, feelings, and emotions of other women who had breast cancer. I needed to hear this to confirm that I was not out of my mind or being dramatic. But you will only meet these women here and there along the way. You can't find them. They seem to find you.

Waiting is the hardest thing to do with a cancer diagnosis.

WORDS CAN HURT OR HEAL, WHAT DID YOURS DO TODAY?

You are in disbelief.

You are hurt.

You are angry.

You are devastated.

You are mad.

All of those emotions are a roller coaster.

And you may not yet have a complete diagnosis.

Not only did my medical institution make me wait three weeks for the blasted biopsy, when the pathologies came back they were not complete. I knew they were estrogen and progesterone positive, but I would "know the HER2 results in just a few days." In order to avoid chemotherapy, I would have to be HER2 negative and no invasion to the lymph nodes; but, the lymph node answer would not be known until the lumpectomy.

The thought of chemotherapy and losing my hair was terrifying. It was more than I could handle. It terrified me beyond words; beyond explanation. I would later hear, I was not alone with this fear either. I would later hear of one chemotherapy patient who never looked in the mirror during her treatments. I would later read about women who also found losing their hair very traumatic. Have you ever heard these stories and fears? These were not the stories that were passed along to me from the "friends and neighbors."

I would also later learn from other breast cancer patients that, from initial mammogram to biopsy results can easily be within a two-week window. Some women, I learned, had their initial mammogram, secondary mammogram, biopsy, and diagnosis within seven days. Others had their cancer diagnosis in 48 hours. One friend had a mammogram on Friday and biopsy three days later on Monday.

I will never know why I had to wait three weeks for a biopsy. It was winter here; the snow birds had gone south. I will never know why I had to wait a total of 17 days for pathology reports while most women wait less than 7. Just bad, bad luck.

Before you go for the biopsy, don't be afraid to pick up that phone for yourself and ask if labs are done on premises or farmed out. Many facilities have complete in-house laboratories, but many don't. So, help your friend or family member and think for them. Anticipate for them. Make the call for them and ask the questions. Something for everyone to consider.

Doctors and nurses along the way would say to me, "You are not going to die from this." At first, I didn't know that. How could I? I never even thought I was at risk for breast cancer. The anxiety that all of this caused me nearly did kill me. I found the waiting to be very, very cruel. It's the not knowing. I think most people would agree that knowing what you are up against is half the battle, but the not knowing can be just too overwhelming. It was for me. I continued to have those terrible dreams and to wake up in the middle of the night in tears.

Of course, I was planning for the worst and hoping for the best, but my world was crashing around me. I was hearing how easy it was for this one. How brave they were. They had the worst diagnosis. Well, let me clear this up for everyone, there is no GOOD cancer diagnosis. Some diagnoses are more complicated than others, but none of them are simple or easy, and by all means, the word *good* just does not apply here. Don't ever let anyone make you feel as though your case is less traumatic than anyone else's. The word cancer is traumatic. Cancer is just a very scary word.

I was still waiting for my HER2 results! I was still waiting for that final diagnosis!

But my wait continued. So, where is that "easy" that I heard so much about?

This begs me to ask the question: If it's so easy, why are there talk shows featuring how one friend supported another through her battle with breast cancer by going with her for every chemotherapy treatment? Or another show that features a woman who has an old high school chum who flew halfway across the country to be there for her friend just after she received her cancer diagnosis?

If it is so easy, then why do you see headlines about movie stars that read; "Opens Up About 'Darkest Days' During Wife's Breast Cancer Battle" or "I didn't know what I was in for" and "It was all so overwhelming"?

And I bet none of these celebrities were worried about punching the time clock or losing their job, house, or car.

I still couldn't wrap my head around how this was possible. I was truly beginning to lose my mind and go MAD!

I actually had one person say to me, "Well, you did smoke cigarettes, and they say that can cause breast cancer." Someone else asked if I had ever used birth control pills. And yet another told me that the sugar in my tea could cause breast cancer. SHUT UP! Believe it or not, your closest confidants will say some of the craziest and sometimes hurtful things.

Your friends and family rally around you with their infinite wisdom when you are facing a medical challenge or any challenge for that matter. Then when the diagnosis is bad news, they begin to sputter pure crap. It doesn't matter whether the diagnosis is breast cancer, scleroderma, lupus, Crohn's disease or any other life-changing diagnosis, they have all the answers. They have that secret little handbook that not even your doctor has.

I venture to say that some of it is a nervous reaction. They don't know what to say, so instead of thinking it through, they just say the first thing that pops into their head. You can imagine how well that works out.

I suspect many do this because never having faced such a diagnosis themselves, they somehow feel they can wish it away. But they can't. Or, I think some must rationalize your diagnosis, justifying why it won't happen to them; "you smoked cigarettes...."

We've all stuck our foot in our mouths, then apologized profusely because we meant no harm or ill-will. But there are other people who say hurtful things. I don't know if it's tough love or a defense mechanism. But why do they do it? Why would a family member tell you after being diagnosed with scleroderma by a doctor that you are a hypochondriac? Why would a friend say you are making a big deal out of breast cancer? More true stories!

Why would people you love or who love you say such things at one of the worst moments in your life? Didn't your mother always tell you to think before you speak? Even if kissing the Blarney Stone was the one and only cause of breast cancer, would you point out last year's vacation and the photo of your loved one kissing the Blarney Stone at such a trying moment in their life? Just saying!

Words really do matter. Words have meaning.

Then I swore my husband to secrecy. I didn't want him to tell the neighbors. I was ashamed. Maybe it was something that I did? Why else would my friends and family have said those things to me? They must be right. It must be my fault, because I have no family history. This shame would continue to haunt me.

What I did learn later was that the most significant risk of breast cancer is being a woman and then age. I can't change who I am, and news flash, none of us are getting any younger. I would also learn that there are contributing factors that might increase the estrogen production that can fuel many breast cancers, such as stress, alcohol, weight gain, and many more. I'm certain every woman could find something on that list and put a big check mark next to it, but these

16

are only possible contributing factors. It is an incredibly basic list. It is unsettling to realize that something as simple as not having children, your evening glass of wine, or those few extra pounds could potentially be a contributing factor. But there are plenty of women who have never gained an ounce, don't drink alcohol and have had children, yet they too are diagnosed with breast cancer.

So, don't think you are immune from breast cancer just because you can't check something off this list. The list is merely possibilities, but being a woman is the biggest risk of all and none of us can really change that. One out of eight ladies, no genes required! Post-menopausal women, it's all about aging and being a woman. I just never knew, did you?

I had a bit of an idea of what might lie ahead in the form of a flyer from my cancer diagnostic center, which was a bit of a road map showing me that, with a HER2-negative diagnosis, I would be treated this way with caveats based on the size of the tumor and what the results were from the surgery. But if HER2 was positive, there would be a completely different treatment plan, of course, with the caveats. I would prefer to go through none of it. All of it was scary.

But a dear friend made it worse and compared me to another friend of hers, and then stated that I was acting like a three-year-old having a temper tantrum by saying "Why me!" Well, hell yeah, why me? None of us deserve this. None of us brought this on ourselves.

I didn't learn or truly understand until later what cancer was— that my cells were improperly dividing and overproducing—or how estrogen and menopause likely could have fueled the cancer.

I'll never forget this same friend telling me how her friend was so brave enduring a double mastectomy, chemotherapy, and radiation. So, I'm not brave because I would prefer to do none of it? Who would look forward to any of this? I'm glad her friend conquered Poseidon, but I'd prefer not to even meet him. Of course, I was distraught. Who wouldn't be? I thought I could confide my deepest and darkest thoughts with my dear friend.

I guess I was wrong.

If all of this is so easy, then why did I read headlines one morning that a celebrity "tells about scare with cancer"? She is making headlines because for 24 hours, ten years ago, she thought she might have cancer. She went on to say how that information ruined the award ceremony she was attending that evening. Yes, it is scary. It ruins many moments, days, and most parts of your life. It can ruin friendships. Very, very scary, particularly when it turns out to be cancer. And this celebrity had to experience her distress for only 24 hours.

The worry and concern and possible shame is hard to get past. Please don't introduce how easy or simple it was for your neighbor. Maybe you don't agree with what your cancer patient is saying or complaining about, but let them express their feelings. They must go through it and live it, you don't.

Just simply say, "I'm sorry this is happening?"

Tell your cancer battler you are there for them. They can call you anytime and you will just listen. I needed someone to just listen. I needed to tell someone about the monsters under my bed. They had no idea how my world was turning upside down. But, my family and close friends should have.

I was just plain scared of what my world would be or could become. Hearing these secondhand stories made it worse. That made it all that much scarier. But no matter which way that HER2 went, the best prognosis would have me undergoing a minimum of 20 radiation treatments. I knew this from the flyer I had been given. Who would look forward to that every single day? Radiation is harmful, right? Who has time for that? I finally asked my friend if her "friend" worked. No, she doesn't. Well then, there you have it, we weren't the same, were we? Having a full-time job where you depend on that income for your car or mortgage payment now has you worrying even more. Maybe your health insurance is through your place of business, too. So please don't compare people. It is just never quite the same. I was scared. I wish my friend could have understood that.

We all have busy lives, and cancer doesn't fit neatly into it for any of us. You, the cancer battler, have the right to feel however you feel. It's hard to understand and accept that your own body has malfunctioned. Nothing genetic here. Nothing you were born with or inherited from your parents. It's okay to be worried. It's okay to be selfish. It's okay to ask, "Why me?" Your body just betrayed and turned on you. It's not your fault.

This disease has wrapped its tentacles around me and is squeezing the life out of me. I don't want to know about them, because this is about me. It has its own design and has set its sights on me.

My bad luck continued, as I had waited another 13 days beyond my cancer diagnosis (which was 17 days after the biopsy) to understand the results of the HER2. It is not unusual for the HER2 to lag a few days after the original cancer diagnosis, but 13 days is quite unusual.

It was 13 days of hell.

In the end, it was March 7th before I knew the final prognosis and treatment plan prescribed for me. I barely slept during the entire month of February and the first week of March. I was completely defeated long before I had a *final prognosis*.

The excessive wait from February 1, 2016, to my final diagnosis on March 7, 2016, beat me down. I continue to struggle with that mental anguish. To worry about dying, harsh treatment, and quality of life for that long was just cruel. It has left its scars on me.

I still do not understand what took so long. Where is the easy, I had heard so much about?

I suppose people say the darnedest things because they don't know what to say. Well, maybe it is time to learn.

A gentleman from my soccer club, summed it up best one day, "I can't even begin to imagine being told I have cancer."

FRIENDS ARE PEOPLE WHO MAKE YOUR PROBLEMS THEIR PROBLEMS SO YOU DON'T HAVE TO GO THROUGH IT ALONE

It was Monday, March 7th. I will never forget the call that kept me from becoming institutionalized. The final pathology was back. I was HER2-negative. That was the best news I could have received. My tumor was considered small, 7mm. I was estrogen/progesterone positive and now we finally knew that I was HER2-negative. I was stage 1, level 2. My tumor was caught very early. This information and the rest would indicate that it had not metastasized, but that was as much as we knew until the lumpectomy.

Finally, I had confirmation of what should be a positive outlook. Chemotherapy should not be part of my future.

Others are not as fortunate. There are so many tentacles to breast cancer that I couldn't even begin to list all the possibilities. A breast cancer patient may not know their complete prognosis until the lumpectomy is complete, or maybe even several days following the lumpectomy.

With breast cancer, the pathologies regarding estrogen, progesterone, and HER2 will dictate your treatment for the most part. It is my understanding that my health care facility outsourced some of these pathologies, specifically the HER2. I had drawn the short straw, again. Wait until there is a full box of specimens before shipping them to another lab for testing. I guess I was the first one in that new box. I had interviewed three different surgeons without that final pathology report. Based on what we knew so far, it would likely come back with a more positive prognosis. However, I learned a long time ago not to assume. I have been down this crazy medical rabbit hole before.

I was interviewing surgeons without the final pathology report. But what was I supposed to do, wait longer? I'm not throwing my institution under the bus, but maybe they need to make some changes. Some women I know had their answers within 48 hours while others waited a full week. I waited and waited with no communication from the breast care center. Maybe women should be preselecting their mammogram facilities based on how they process a possible cancer patient's pathologies. Hindsight is interesting, something to consider.

Some women learn after their lumpectomies that the cancer has metastasized. In other words, it has moved to other parts of the body and the cancer had invaded elsewhere. Others learn that the entire tumor was removed with clear margins and you are ready to move on to the next stage. While others may have to return for a second lumpectomy because clear margins were not obtained. And some women must go through chemotherapy before anything can be done because their tumor is so large and aggressive.

Where is the simple and easy in all of that?

Why would friends, family, nurses, and doctors tell you not to worry when this is what you could be up against? Why do doctors and nurses paint pretty pictures of pink ponies and unicorns? I realize they need to supply hope, but I need reality. I suppose they are trying to be upbeat and positive. Please, give it to me straight! It needs to be understood what a breast cancer patient is expected to endure.

There are many steps to breast cancer treatment with various possibilities. Radiation can be 16 or 40 visits. Chemotherapy could come before a lumpectomy and/or after the lumpectomy. Some women must endure chemotherapy, surgery, chemotherapy, and then radiation. There's always a next step, and the steps are different for each person. And it never seems to end. The statement "piece of cake" is not synonymous with Chemotherapy or Radiation. None of these treatments are easy; not for anyone no matter what they tell you.

And all you do is worry every step of the way.

When that first blip on the mammography screen occurs, it cannot tell anyone what the final story will be. When that first "blip" occurs, everyone should bite their tongues because the true answers are just not known, not yet. If you are speaking with someone who has just been diagnosed with breast cancer, or is waiting for their diagnosis, please choose your words carefully. Will you be sitting there with them when their 1 P.M, 15-minute treatment is now pushed back to 3:30 P.M.? Will you drop them at the door when the rain is falling harshly and there is no place to park? Please keep all of this in mind when you are telling someone "don't worry" or "it won't be cancer."

So, how will you help?

Will you go to the pharmacy for ointment when their skin is peeling from the radiation? Will you take time off from work and sit by your friend's side week after week or month after month during chemotherapy treatment? Will you shave your head when your sister's beautiful red curls fall out? Will you walk their dog when radiation has them completely exhausted? Will you hold your cousin's head over the toilet following chemotherapy treatments? Be supportive, but never offer false hope. Please remember, you told them not to worry. You told them it wouldn't be cancer.

I had nearly lost my mind and couldn't understand why no one else thought this was a big deal. Surgery, radiation, and drug therapy is a big deal. And don't forget, enduring 36 days of not knowing if chemotherapy was going to be prescribed. The drug therapies are meant to reduce recurrence. So, there you go, it can come back. Did you know that?

One of the nurses who delivered all the information to me pointed out that she had been through breast cancer twice. Yikes! Did I need to know that? Where is the simple in all of this? I began to think there was something wrong with me? Why do I feel so lost and scared? Why am I the only one to find this all so horrendous?

Women are strong, and we plow through most challenges because that is just what we do! We persevere. Pile it on—work, children, activities, household—we'll get through! We can always handle one more thing. Is that why I was hearing, "It was easy for my friend" or "It was simple for my neighbor"? But this was just one challenge too many for me.

I know, what choice is there, but that is also the rub. You have no control. You are a puppet on a string that has a million other obligations and aspirations and you are no longer in control of your time, mind or body.

Why was I expected to look forward to all of this? Why was I expected to look forward to all of this with a smile? Why was I told I needed a better attitude because I was so much better off than so many others? More true stories!

I knew the medical challenges that I could be facing. I knew what I could be up against; my family and friends didn't.

As long as I have my 34-C's, the return of breast cancer is quite real.

I needed to hit bottom and find my fight, not be held up with false hope and unrealistic expectations. I needed to grieve. The diagnosis, prognosis and long-term effects are traumatic no matter what anyone tells you. As crazy as it sounds, I needed to hit bottom and grieve, and for my family to grieve with me, to find my fight; because you are always looking over your shoulder for it to rear its ugly head again.

Instead, I began to shut down and keep it all to myself. My friends and family just didn't understand how scared and afraid I was of what life could become. I wondered if other women had similar experiences to mine and chose to say little or nothing. Thus, I shout again from the rooftops!

Maybe other women too felt looked down upon. People look at you as though it is your fault. It's something you did or caused yourself. Some actually said just that. I felt a sense of shame throughout all of this. Maybe other women didn't share their true feelings or stories with friends and family after all. Maybe they didn't want to be seen as vulnerable. Or maybe other women, too, experienced what I did. Maybe they, too, kept it to themselves in the end.

I have since learned that it is completely unreasonable to expect someone to be fearless in the face of cancer. You need to be able to express your fears honestly. Avoiding these emotions is potentially harmful. There is nothing wrong with the feelings and emotions that you experience. Because you are frightened, scared or worried does not mean there is something wrong with you. It does not mean that you are broken.

I remember when my children were babies. I found the infant and toddler stage to be quite challenging. I was tired and unhappy with motherhood. Yet all I would hear from my friends was how wonderful everything was with motherhood. Everything was perfect! I thought, what was wrong with me? Then I met a woman who would tell me that people never quite tell the whole truth. They never want to show their shortcomings or vulnerabilities, even your best friends. She then went on to give me some advice that I never forgot: "You will always love your children, but there will be some days that you don't like them very much." In other words, it was okay to feel as though life isn't a bed of roses, because it isn't.

I guess I always thought I could be brutally honest with my closest confidants. There were less than a handful of people I was confiding in. They didn't like what I had to say.

Looking back now, I think my friend was right!

JUST BECAUSE ONE PERSON'S PROBLEM IS LESS TRAUMATIC THAN ANOTHER'S DOESN'T MEAN THEY ARE REQUIRED TO HURT LESS

Surgery finally came on March 14th. This was 77 days after the initial mammogram when the anomaly was seen. I had a wonderful surgeon who paved the way for me. I had only met her on March 4th, but she made me feel as though I was the most important patient she had.

I'm glad I took the time to interview multiple surgeons. Living near a large city does have its benefits. It made me feel a bit more in control.

A lumpectomy is a simpler surgery than a mastectomy, but the anxiety of it all is overwhelming. After all, you are under anesthesia. There are many germs in hospitals and there are plenty of horror stories to keep you up at night about those germs. Despite it being the best possible diagnosis, it is still scary and overwhelming and very time-consuming.

After an hour-and-a-half drive, I arrived at the hospital for my surgery. I was told to be there for an 11:30 check-in and I would be sent straight to radiology. I arrived shortly after 11 a.m. I don't like to be late. They checked me in rather quickly and sent me to radiology where I was told my appointment wasn't until 12:30; just over an hour from now. Imagine my surprise, no one had mentioned an "appointment" for radiology. So please sit and wait. Lovely!

When they finally called me, sometime well after 12:30 p.m., the technician explained that while I sat in this oversized chair, with my breast being compressed in the mammogram machine, they would be inserting a guidewire. She kindly explained this after prefacing that she had never personally experienced it, then asked me how that sounded. I found that question odd, because it all sounded terrifying to me. Wire? Additionally, she explained that they would be injecting dye so that the surgeon could find the lymph nodes. For some unknown reason, which should have been a red flag for me since my biopsy was simple, she found it necessary to state that most people find the biopsy more challenging than the dye, but the dye could produce a *slight* burn. WELL, SHE WAS WRONG! When the dye was injected, I nearly hit the ceiling. Tears flowed uncontrollably down my cheeks due to an extreme burning sensation. The radiologist hugged me. He could see my distress.

When I emerged from radiology, my husband took one look at me and asked what was wrong.

As if all of this wasn't challenging enough, I'm now in a hospital gown with a wire hanging from my breast, and they ask me if I want to put my regular cloths back on, or would I prefer to walk across the parking lot in my hospital gown. Sure, let me put my bra back on and I'll just flop that wire to the side!! And, by the way, there is no bridge or walkway back to the main building. This is March. It's back out into the cold, rainy weather while dodging cars exiting the parking garage. There must be a better way!

My hat's off to the nurses and caregivers in these hospitals, but they too must choose their words carefully. While I was in pre-op, a nice young man who I believe was a nurse asked me how things went in radiology regarding the guidewire. Before I could answer, he further stated, "Piece of cake, right?" If I hadn't been hooked up to an IV I might have strangled him. I looked him right in the eyes and asked, "When was the last time you had that done? It was the worst pain I have ever experienced in my life." He sheepishly smiled and responded, "Ahhh, you have a point."

Walking across the cold parking lot in my "johnny" was humiliating. I felt like cattle going to slaughter. Not all lumpectomy patients have to walk across parking lots dodging cars, but I do know there are many other stories just like this that could be inserted here. I have heard stories from other cancer patients that you would not believe and that would leave you shaking your head. No wonder we keep it to ourselves. No one would believe us.

I'm not trying to embarrass my hospital. If the cancer returns I will use this institution and surgeon again. I have great respect for them. I'm just pointing out that none of it is easy. You, our friends and family of supporters, have no idea what we may be subjected to and expected to endure.

Just a little dignity, please!

I was trying to remain positive throughout all of this, but geez, the curveballs kept coming. I began to look in the mirror and question what I did to deserve all of this. Could I just catch one break, please? Ok, at least it wasn't snowing when I had to cross that parking lot in my "johnny."

There are a lot of feelings and emotions, and some people want to talk. I did. And I didn't want to talk to strangers. I had read on the Internet where one woman said, "Well, why not me? I've had a good life and I can handle it." I could see it now, a room full of strangers at some support meeting and all of them saying they deserved it. Oh, heaven help me. I know I didn't deserve this and I don't think anyone does. But ladies, here's the dirty little secret. You are at risk because you are a woman, and that risk increases as you age. Lovely!

This begins to take a toll on your family, too. Not only was there no handbook for me, but there wasn't one for them, either. I can't imagine having younger, school-age children through all of this, because this was very hard on my adult children, too. My emotions were wild. I was more than defeated before I even had my final diagnosis let alone before any treatment had begun. I had already lost the will to fight that I normally would have had. I never thought of it until later, but I believe it was hard for them to see their strong mother, who could tackle anything, coming apart.

But, for 36 days, I imagined losing my hair, being sicker than sick from chemotherapy, and the possibility of cancer returning again and again. Or worse! I know the doctors and nurses said I was not going to die from this, but they also told me not to worry. They told me my risk was small. They were wrong. My experience showed me they haven't been right so far, so what has changed now? It was just too much. All of this just became too much for me to handle.

I later would learn of a high school friend battling breast cancer for a second time. My worry was warranted.

Your friends and relatives text you and say hooray, all went well and that's the last you hear from most of them. Hindsight, maybe they ran because it was hard on them, too. But some of them were never there to begin with. That made me sad.

Sometimes there are complications! I know one cancer patient who ended up with an awful rash from the tape that was used during her lumpectomy. Another cancer patient had her lumpectomy, then had to go back for a second lumpectomy as her surgeon did not get clear margins. And yet another developed a seroma, so her first radiation treatment was delayed by a several weeks to allow this to resolve. Then there are those who learn the cancer has invaded the lymph nodes and invaded other parts of the body. Chemotherapy is now needed. It just goes on and on. Nothing simple here!

These are just a few perfect examples as to why you should choose your words wisely and not offer false hope. These are perfect examples why breast cancer patients continue to need support. There is always another challenge. There is always another side-effect that no one mentioned. But know, a smiley face in their email inbox saying I'm here to help, could make a difference. Ask how you could help.

The breast cancer treatment regimen can be a virtual marathon. Some marathons are shorter than others, but they are all long. By no means is the treatment over just because you had a lumpectomy. The surgery isn't the end, however. It's just the beginning.

SOME PEOPLE CAN MAKE YOU LAUGH A LITTLE LOUDER AND SMILE A LITTLE BRIGHTER

I knew that my next step would be radiation. The thought of radiation was scary. There is a reason that when you have an X-ray at the dentist, which is a lower dose of radiation, they cover you with a lead jacket and the technician leaves the room. It was hard to wrap my mind around subjecting myself to what most would consider harmful.

But before you can begin, please sign here; left breast radiation could cause a heart attack. Lovely, that's me! And please sign there; radiation could cause new cancers. Seriously?

I learned that I would need to go to the local hospital every day for 20 visits for radiation "therapy" after 3 visits to "set-up." Oh, but wait. You can't start for another 6 weeks. What? I'm looking to get my life back to normal. I am looking to put this in my rearview mirror and that is just not an option. Apparently, you need to have additional healing time following the surgery before you are subjected to the radiation. That makes sense. But this just won't go away. When I expressed my displeasure with this new life schedule, I heard, "It will be over before you know it," "Piece of cake," and "No big deal."

I was finally tired of hearing all of these platitudes.

I challenged my supporters to pick a time in the middle of their day and go stand in a corner for 15 minutes at the exact same time each day. You don't even have to leave your office! I stated that I bet they couldn't complete 3 days of this challenge. To date, I know of no one who accepted my challenge.

This would consume my entire month of May.

Traffic begins to increase during the spring in my little tourist town. The kids will soon be out of school, but I'm still dodging school buses and need to allow myself at least 30 and sometimes 45 minutes to get to my hospital. Then add a bit more time to park and to get changed. It wasn't always easy finding a parking spot, either, and on the rainy days, the available spots were farthest from the door. It can be very raw here in May, particularly on rainy days. A valet service is available at my hospital; however, on rainy days they were always terribly backed up. I just couldn't leave work any earlier than I already had. And remember, I live in a small town!

For more than 5 weeks, each and every day I went to the hospital all by myself.

Then you wait. All in all, this would consume nearly 2 hours of my day, Monday through Friday over a 5-week period. No big deal, right?

During all of this, I listened to friends and family complain about cheerleading practice being changed from 3 to 4 o'clock; "that doesn't fit into my schedule." Or the soccer game was moved from this field to that field; "terribly inconvenient." Or the boss canceled a meeting at the last moment and I sat in horrendous traffic to get there. For some reason, everyone else is permitted to complain about the inconveniences they are experiencing, but breast cancer patients are not. I suppose what other choice is there, but therein lies the rub.

Please understand, just because it's cancer doesn't mean, we too can't become overwhelmed with this world of inconvenience.

Then I became concerned about my job. I was in sales and had goals to meet. It was a new company for me, and I was worried. I had a very supportive boss, but that doesn't always help you keep your job. I heard from family that they would never fire me over this. Well, folks, I have news for you. Do some research and you will find all sorts of support groups and websites out there that are dedicated to helping those who have been dismissed from their jobs due to cancer treatments. Later, I would learn that my concerns came to fruition for someone else in my company. Funny, I had every right to be worried.

I also learned from my research that despite the harm radiation can do, this would reduce my risk of recurrence by 50%. Nothing comes without consequences, however. There are side effects to radiation. They give you a little brochure warning you that this could cause a severe sunburn. Oh, joy! This could cause itching, rash, and dry skin. How fun! This can cause fatigue. I'm already tired! And if you have any issues, to call your radiation oncologist.

I have a foot doctor who always tells me that it is hard to invoke pain on yourself, referring to having an ingrown toenail removed. He says that's why people come to see him. Day 1 down, 19 more days of treatment ahead. It is hard to look forward to this no matter how helpful it would be.

Still looking for simple and easy…. but I digress.

But I would keep my chin up and endure all of this, including the humiliation I felt with each appointment. There I sat in a waiting area that was a glorified busy hallway with men old enough to be my great-grandfather. All of us in our little "johnny's" hoping nothing is hanging out. The door to the lobby waiting area was always open, so anyone could see who was sitting there waiting for treatment. No privacy. It was very awkward. Then they would take you into a room, and sometimes your technicians were two men, which I found uncomfortable. So, your arms are over your head and your feet are loosely bound and your breasts are hanging out. Oh, please just a little dignity!

Sometimes, equipment breaks down and you must wait for the repair technician to arrive and repair the equipment, so now your appointment is hours after its originally scheduled time. Or maybe they reschedule your appointment for another day entirely. So, you must just adjust and squeeze this into your already full schedule. There are no choices here. That light at the end of the tunnel moves on you. Your last day of treatment is no longer May 23rd. This just adds to your concern about job security.

It is impossible to plan for anything.

I followed the instructions and dutifully lathered myself with aloe following treatments, before bed, and after my shower. Just about halfway through the treatments, I found myself more tired than usual, and I was generally asleep by 8 P.M. each night. I would sleep a good 10 hours most nights. I drank plenty of water to stay well-hydrated, to the point I thought I was going to drown. I noticed that my breast was swollen, and I continued to wear the sports bra for fear of popping right out of a regular bra, and my shirt, and shock the world! I began to itch a bit heading into my final week of treatment. I only had to endure 20 treatments. I can't even imagine going through what some do at 40 treatments.

None of this is easy or a piece of cake. It is a long, long road and it still isn't over. If only my friends and family had asked how they could help, but they didn't. They just didn't know what I was going through. They don't know what women are expected to endure. But they never asked either.

It would have been nice to come home to a greeting card in my mailbox that just said, "thinking of you." A simple smiley face in my inbox when I got home would have helped. Maybe not to have to cook dinner one evening could have given me a bit of extra energy.

You will meet and reconnect with other breast cancer battlers along the way. Another old high school friend summed it up best during her final week of radiation treatment. Simply put, "I just can't wait for it to be over."

It's far from over.

SOME DAYS YOU ARE THE DOG AND SOME DAYS YOU ARE THE HYDRANT

I have had quite a few medical challenges most recently. I had finally gotten back on my feet; a new job with possibly a great career ahead of me. That's why this hit me that much harder and really knocked me on my butt.

Recently, a former co-worker told me that he had a cousin who had just been diagnosed. He asked me what he could do for her. He told me that he wanted her to know that he was there for her if she wanted to talk. She didn't want to talk at this point and he didn't understand. Funny, some people want to talk and talk, and others don't. I told him, just keep reminding her that you are available. Send her a card. Take her to lunch. Send her flowers. Take her out for coffee. Just check in on her. Ask her how she is doing and ask what you can do to help. Just let her know you are there and that you care. Don't let her feel forgotten, alone or abandoned.

Support will come from places when you least expect it. I ran into a former coworker while getting coffee, and I told her about the cancer diagnosis. She stayed in touch with me and texted me here and there over the next few months to see if she could be of help, or to ask if I needed anything. A true friend.

I had another coworker text me out of the blue offering to drive me home from radiation in the event I was too tired.

My new office sent me the most beautiful flowers following my surgery.

I received a greeting card from my sister's friend. I have only met her a few times. Another friend of my sister called to offer her support. She is a cancer survivor.

One business associate looked at me and said, "I'm sorry you have to go through this." That meant the world to me. It is a lonely time with many fears and side effects. It is important to know that people do care and that you are not alone.

Along the way, I met a wonderful woman. I think she might have been my angel. She told me something that I would repeat to myself for months. It helped me. She said, "Life is what happens while you are busy making other plans." I would learn later that this quote, attributed to Allen Saunders, was a line John Lennon used in his song "Beautiful Boy." But this stranger, who was actually a potential client, continued to check on me. She offered to take me to my treatments. I had only just met her. We barely knew one another. She is a cancer survivor.

What surprised me the most was who didn't call, text, email, or send flowers or ask how they could help.

I was through surgery and radiation, and this all should now be in my rearview mirror. But it wasn't. Something was nagging at me. A dear friend was able to put her finger on what was haunting me: "We are all just in remission."

That's it! For the first time in my adult life, I've realized my own mortality.

This is cancer—a common, survivable disease but one that can bite you in the ass again at any time. Cancer is a mysterious disease. If it happened once, what is to keep it from happening again?

Sadly, it does recur for way too many. That's why they say, "You are cancer-free." They never tell you that you are cured. There is no cure.

Some people have a lifetime to adjust growing up with asthma, Crohn's disease, cystic fibrosis, diabetes, lupus, or even peanut allergies. I'm sure it was a hard adjustment when first diagnosed. Why wouldn't adjusting to breast cancer be hard, too? It doesn't go away just because you had surgery and treatments. It can happen again and again. Just ask my friend who was diagnosed a second time. It can lie in remission waiting to blindside you years from now. That's just plain mean! Read the statistics for yourself regarding rates of recurrence. They, too, increase with age. This is a huge concern to me, and I want everyone to hear this LOUD & CLEAR! Know this! Don't be blindsided like I was.

I tell you this next part in detail because, as I noted earlier, I have been down this medical rabbit hole before. My experience told me that nothing is ever the way it appears to be. It's all a long road with twists and turns. Things happen, and things go wrong.

One day, I had a sore spot on my fingertip. Long story short, after seven months of going from PCP to specialists to wound care, a cuticle issue that would deteriorate under a doctor's care would become infected from a grocery cart or countertop, I was told, and left me with my right index finger one-quarter inch shorter.

A few months later, I began to have pain in my right leg. Over the next year and a half, I went from doctor to doctor—seven all told. I saw some of them multiple times. There were many tests and much physical therapy, yet no one knew what was wrong. I gave up sports officiating. I could barely walk halfway down the aisle of the grocery store due to severe pain. I couldn't even walk the dog to the mailbox. The pain was debilitating.

Finally, when my big toe began to turn black, they figured out my debilitating pain was due to something called claudication, which is a lack of blood flow in the leg. The femoral artery in my right leg was completely occluded, but they were uncertain why. Maybe a blood clot? My doctor was going to open my artery with a stent and I would be all better. Well, he couldn't, so an arterial bypass was in my future. He told me, "We lost some of your toe, but we saved your foot and leg, for now." But that surgery failed within 90 days.

This surgeon emphatically stated, he did not want to operate again. He told me some pills would help me walk with a bit less pain. Oh, really? Now how is that possible? It couldn't before, what is different now? The blood flow to my leg was minimal. I had visions of a simple auto accident causing trauma, and I would end up losing my foot or leg due to this lack of blood flow.

We had to start over, and a year later a new surgeon performed another bypass. Allowing for a two-hour drive every 30, 60 then 90 days, my new surgeon monitored me closely. I spent the next year and a half on Warfarin. I went every week or two for blood tests due to the Warfarin. I went so often that it became very painful each time they inserted the needle to draw blood. More than a year had now passed and the bypass was still a success. I had thought my luck had changed.

I was wrong again.

So, you see, this hit me particularly hard. I have faced, "next time we may have to amputate your finger." I have faced, "we saved your foot and leg, for now." I'm not trying to be melodramatic. I've had my share of hurdles. My close friends and family know all of this. But, I know how things can go wrong. I've experienced what can go wrong first hand.

Along the way, I learned that cancer can cause blood clots. It made me wonder. I will be doubly looking over my shoulder going forward.

I was now feeling targeted. When is it going to end, and how? I couldn't help but think of the movie, *Final Destination*. Was it coming for me no matter what? My mind became a very scary place.

I know life isn't fair, but geez, when is it going to cut me a break? Why not just strike me with a bolt of lightning?

Yes, I did feel sorry for myself.

In my opinion, I'm allowed!

You, too, are allowed. Those who tell you otherwise have not walked in these shoes.

I wanted to talk. I needed to talk. I needed someone to tell me the monsters were no longer under my bed; if only they could. Eventually, I would speak to a very nice social worker. It helped. But I didn't want to talk to a stranger, especially not in the beginning. I began to keep a journal. I found writing helped me express my emotions.

I would later find a blogger who had a way with words. It was so refreshing to read. She writes, "It's ok to be selfish." I needed to read and hear this. I still do. You need to know you are not alone. You need to know that other cancer patients have the same thoughts, feelings, and crazy experiences that you do. But you don't find it easily while you are going through all of this. You find it later.

So, you see, I was feeling lower than low. I was tired and sore. Radiation treatments will stay with you. I was told I would continue to be tired four to six weeks after my final treatment, and I was for a good eight weeks. And I see my radiation oncologist again six months after my last treatment. There must be a reason for these additional visits, otherwise, why would I continue to have follow-up visits with a radiation oncologist? So, my marathon must not yet be complete.

A greeting card or text message would have been helpful at this point. I would have loved a flower or a call. I don't think the average person realizes how extensive and time consuming the simplest case of breast cancer can be. It invades your life and takes over. You can't even begin to imagine how you must juggle these appointments and still fit work and life into your day. You might as well have taken on another full-time job.

Have you ever noticed upon entering a store or your bank you are greeted with, "How are you today?" You walk into work and co-workers say, "Good morning, how are you?" So why does no one call, text, or email you to ask that same question while you are undergoing cancer treatments? Are they afraid of the answer? Or maybe they just don't realize how important it is to ask the questions.

It would have been nice to hear from anyone just to know I still had a support system. It would have been nice to not feel so alone. It would have been nice to have been asked.

It would have been nice to not feel forgotten.

YOU WILL NEVER TRULY UNDERSTAND SOMETHING UNTIL IT HAPPENS TO YOU

That brings me to the next phase of treatment—oral medications. For the five years following your diagnosis and treatment, most women will be prescribed a daily dose of tamoxifen (used mostly for those who have not gone through menopause) or an aromatase inhibitor. When used for cancer treatment, aromatase inhibitors—Femara and Arimidex—are generally prescribed to those who have experienced menopause.

Just like all the evening commercials that we see with endless side effects, the aromatase inhibitors have a long list of issues, too. Bone loss, hot flashes, joint pain, night sweats, fatigue, swelling, and weight gain are just a few of the nicer known side effects. The list goes on. My neighbor would tell me how her mother-in-law just completed her five years of the aromatase inhibitors, and she feels her bones are now so brittle that they could snap at any moment.

I didn't need to know that.

What next?

I began my aromatase inhibitor, Femara, in mid-August. After about a week, I began to feel tired. In short order, I became exceptionally tired with a bit of nausea. I inquired with the pharmacist and was advised that the body will adjust within about three weeks. Then the dizziness began. By the end of the first 30 days, it was all

I could do not to walk over to the sofa and curl up and sleep. I felt like I was on sleeping pills around the clock. I forged ahead and kept trying. I tried to take this medication at dinnertime hoping the side effects would be less intrusive during the daytime. Finally, one day at 2 P.M. while standing in a store, I had to grab two clothing racks because the dizziness was so overwhelming. I thought for sure I was going to be sitting on the floor in short order.

That had not been my first extreme dizzy spell. The week before, I became so dizzy in the grocery aisle that I stood there hanging on to the grocery cart for dear life while leaning against the freezer to keep myself from falling to the floor. These were not isolated incidents, either. There were others. I was woozy and the room would waver for me each morning during my one-mile treadmill workout, my safety net for that previously failed arterial bypass surgery.

As if feeling catatonic and dizzy most of the time wasn't enough, the swelling and soreness were still there for me. I consulted with my radiation oncologist and he prescribed edema therapy. He did say my swelling was unusual. Lucky me! Two days per week I would go to the local physical therapy center for a type of massage therapy. I was grateful to have this opportunity. It did help, but just one more side effect that needed a set date and time to help undo the damage. It was hard to get a consistent appointment schedule as well. I don't know how others can leave work at odd and different hours of the day for such therapy.

At this point, I finally took a leave of absence from work so that I could manage all of this. Many full-time jobs and even some part-time jobs could never accommodate all of these appointments.

Come October, my oncologist prescribed Arimidex instead of Femara. After seven days, I felt good. I said to my husband, "I think this one is going to work." At day 10, I felt like I had the flu. This was now mid-October, so indeed, maybe I was coming down with something. I then developed a cough. I had a pressure on my chest that felt like I was coming down with bronchitis. A bit of fatigue began. I began to take my temperature daily. It was normal. As I approached the third week with no signs of fever, I stopped taking the medication. About five days later, the symptoms went away, so I tried to take the medication again. Ten days later, flu-like symptoms had returned.

What made this all the more challenging was if you mentioned these side-effects to anyone, they looked at you like you were telling a tale! Recently, one old high school friend began to experience night sweats, hair loss, fatigue and more. When she telephoned her oncologist's office she was told that hair loss, night sweats and fatigue were not side effects to this medication. But they are; check FDA.gov. Why does no one talk about this? Why is this information buried and not on those evening commercials?

These oral medications are meant to reduce the recurrence risk. Aromatase inhibitors work by inhibiting the action of the enzyme aromatase, which converts androgens into estrogens. The alternative to the AIs is Tamoxifen, which works to decrease the effects of estrogen produced by the body. According to my oncologist, when you inhibit your body's normal events, you can get side effects. This is true of all medications

Not everyone experiences such severe side effects. Some experience none. But all you hear is how this neighbor and friend took those medications without any issue at all.

So, what is wrong with me?

The day before Thanksgiving, my oncologist suggested I try Tamoxifen instead. I was two for two in the side effect department. I expected my oncologist to suggest Tamoxifen, so I did my research before my appointment. A well-known side effect of Tamoxifen is uterine cancer. Another known side effect is blood clots. From what I read, blood clots to the lungs are most significant, but the entire body can also be affected. Taking Tamoxifen would have reduced my risk of recurring breast cancer from 5.5% to 2.75% for the next five years, but it would give me a 4.75% chance of uterine cancer. My grandmother died of uterine cancer. Something I had discovered during all of this.

My oncologist explained they have a strict protocol and would monitor me closely while taking Tamoxifen. There must be a reason for these extra precautions, right? In addition to seeing him every 90 days, they would monitor me with additional testing, such as ultrasounds and more. He went on to say that worst case, they would perform a complete hysterectomy. Hysterectomy?

Like my foot doctor said, it's hard to invoke pain on yourself. I wasn't willing to accept the risk of blood clots with my vascular history. I wasn't feeling lucky about uterine cancer, either. Luck has not been on my side so far. I decided I was not willing to trade one cancer for another.

I can't live with the flu for the next five years nor can I risk falling in stores over the next five years. A hard decision to make, but the side effects were too severe for me. I'm not alone, as many studies show that 25% to 50% of women stop taking these medications due to the side effects (Mammography, 2016). The present protocol is for five years. I am now reading that 10 years may be the new protocol. You can read it all for yourself at FDA.gov.

So, you see, this is never over. I thought long and hard about trying the Tamoxifen, too! I feverishly poured over trial programs. I learned from a colleague that surgery was required to undo the harm the Tamoxifen had done to her. I consulted my urogynecologist and she did admit that she performs hysterectomies due to cancer from Tamoxifen.

Finally, I was meeting and speaking with other women and heard first hand their experience with side-effects. I am not the only one to experience adverse side-effects. I am not the only one to stop taking these medications. I'm sorry they do not have this "safety net," either. As selfish as it sounds, it is utterly reassuring to know that you are not alone. It was reassuring to know that it's not all just in my head. It is a reality whether anyone believes you or not. But why does no one talk about these side-effects?

I'm sorry to keep asking, but where is the "simple and no big deal" in all of this?

So, I took control of the information and made the best decision for me. I made a very informed and well-thought-out decision. One I'm willing to live with.

However, no one can make these decisions for you. There is no one to speak to, either. The professionals can only offer you the statistics, but you must make your decisions alone. That, too, adds to your stress, fear, and pressure level.

Should the cancer ever return, I will always wonder. You see, none of this will ever go away.

Early November, I remember hearing the disappointment in my sister's voice when I told her I had to stop these medications. I know that she is worried, but I'm worried, too. Personally, I should not have been driving while taking those aromatase inhibitors, so how would I get to work? I've made my decision and am finally taking control of the uncontrollable.

I can live with that! But I will always be looking over my shoulder.

THE NEW NORMAL

Radiation therapy was now in my rearview mirror. I was adjusting to my "new normal."

Months later, the radiated breast still swollen and looking a bit lopsided, I began to experience a "pins & needles" sensation as I approached the end of my workday. Gravity was not my friend. If I leaned forward, the pressure I felt was quite uncomfortable because my "34'C" felt like a bowling ball about ready to fall out and go kerplunk.

And then there are the long-term effects of radiation. A year later my breast is sore to the touch in spots, firm, swollen and feeling bruised. Nothing gets near these 34-C's so how could it possibly be bruised?

Then there are those hugs you get for birthdays, holidays and special occasions and you just cringe through them, because it's painful. I again inquired with my radiation oncologist and yes, these are normal experiences. I checked my pile of brochures; none mentioned that *hugging could be hazardous*!

I checked all of my lists and none told me to take two aspirin when my "34-C" gets a headache. Nor does it mention my yoga days are over because I can no longer lie face down on the floor due to this "new normal." And I'm certain the word lopsided was not printed on any handout, brochure or pamphlet; I checked!

I checked in with my old friend who was diagnosed a few months after me. I told her about my "new normal" and she replied, "mine too is achy & tingly sometimes. I thought I was going nuts....". I guess she missed that paragraph on her brochures as well!

Despite knowing my friend is experiencing just what I am, your mind plays with you. I was certain the cancer was back, so I visited my surgeon. Yes, this is all quite normal and I can expect it to be this way for 2 years, 10 years or possibly forever. I am certain the words forever were not printed anywhere. I looked!

I re-read those endless brochures and pamphlets that I had been given in the beginning. Yes, they mention *slight swelling* and firmness, but I wished they had listed, "Caution during hugs!"

Why do doctors and nurses paint pretty pictures of pink ponies and unicorns? I realize they need to supply hope but I need reality. Tell me my sports bra will be my best friend for the next few years! Give it to me straight! Give me all of the rare examples, because I always seem to be that "exception"!

I think at the end of any treatment they need to hand you a card that fits into your wallet that reads, and the fine prints says, *don't be surprised if.......*

THERE IS A RAINBOW SOMEWHERE AFTER EACH RAIN STORM!

While attempting to make the best decisions, and feeling awful due to aromatase inhibitors and the "new normal," I came upon a sign that read "Making Strides against Breast Cancer Walk," and noted that this walk was coming to my community in late October. Could this be what I needed to feel as though I was finally back in control? Would this help put all of this in my rearview mirror and up on the shelf? I've realized my own mortality and I need to feel in control because my life had been out of control for the past nine months. My husband is getting ready to have his knees replaced. He won't be able to walk with me. Most of my relatives live hundreds of miles away.

I stopped to see someone who I consider a friend. We may not be close confidants and we may not socialize each weekend, but she is a good soul, one I felt I could turn to. She lost both of her parents to cancer. I had forgotten that at the time. I walked into her office and asked if she would participate in the walk with me. She said, "Of course I will." She was my first team member. I cried.

I reached out to friends, coworkers, and former coworkers. A small team, but a wonderful team of good people. People, you can call true friends. Some worried they were too out of shape; others were concerned about the distance, but they stepped up to the plate! I cried!

I thank each and every one of you. You have no idea how tremendously you helped me. I am so very grateful for your incredible support.

It will surprise you who will step up to the plate and who will not. You will feel overjoyed and you will feel sad.

This national organization raises money for cancer research for ALL cancers. When you sign up you create a team and they create a challenge for you to raise money. Raising money is not required, but I thought it was a great diversion for me and, of course, for a great cause. I reached out to family and friends to contribute with a monetary donation. If a monetary contribution was not possible, you could go to the website and post a "cheer" or a "go get 'em" on my webpage.

I'm sorry to say there were a lot of nonresponses. I even went around this National- website and sent out personal invites from my personal email.

CRICKETS!

It wasn't about the money, it was about the support.

The silence made me feel all alone again. How time-consuming could it have been to reply to my email and say, "We hope you have great weather for the walk" or "We wished we could be there with you"? They were just too busy. How very sad.

I suppose it is your real friends who are not too busy. I was too busy for all of this, too, but that was not a choice that I had.

I continued to attempt to keep my chin up and head held high, but the lack of support from those you have personally supported was a sad time for me. It again beat me down.

I recently learned of another business associate who was going through chemotherapy. I couldn't wait to get home and call her to offer a shoulder.

I wished I had known earlier. I could have baked Christmas cookies for her, or helped wrap presents, or driven her to the hospital. I know she has family, but so did I. Maybe just an experienced non-stranger to speak to could have made her day a bit easier. Support!

Just for her to know that someone was there for her and she was not forgotten. Someone was rooting for her!

No one should ever feel alone. Unfortunately, many women do. I've since read this sentiment time and time again in books, articles and blogs. I just wanted to be sure that she never felt that way.

What I think I finally realized is people do not know what to do or say. Their biggest dilemma is what to cook for dinner. So, they say nothing. But, the silence hurts the most. When you need someone the most, they just disappear. It's a scar to your heart and soul. It runs deep and lasts a long, long time.

Therefore, I write my story. It's not about woe is me, it's about what you can do to make a difference. It's about what you can do to help.

Not long after I had finished my radiation therapy, I met with an in-law of my sister for lunch. She calmly stated that she decided to forgo her mammogram for the past two years because she was concerned about the exposure to the radiation. I nearly fell out of my chair.

Well, I sat right up and explained just how grateful I was that I hadn't missed my mammogram and why. If you think that low dose of radiation for a mammogram is something to be concerned about once per year, just you wait till you see the dose of radiation you get with cancer! And depending which little bastard gets you, HER2-positive or HER2-negative in cahoots with ER-positive or ER-negative, you could be visiting that radiation machine for up to 40 times!

And if you think the radiation is a problem, if the cancer is not caught early and/or does metastasize, you get to try the elixir called chemotherapy!

What I've learned is that approximately 85% of breast cancer occurs in women with no family history of breast cancer. This occurs due to genetic mutations that occur because of the aging process rather than inherited mutations. A woman's risk is due to being a woman and getting older. Don't forget, "no genes required."

The radiation from the mammogram is NOTHING compared to cancer therapy radiation or the chemotherapy treatments. And that once a year appointment takes so little time compared to all the cancer radiation and/or chemotherapy appointments.

For now, that big ugly machine is *the* first line of defense for women over 40.

I hope our conversation made a difference in her life. I hope my story makes a difference in your life.

So, don't run from your friends and relatives, embrace them. Make time in your life for them. After all, this could be you, your wife, or your daughter.

Ask how you can help. Ask what you can do. Walk in their shoes and ask yourself, what could I do to make a difference.

Well, I walked that walk—all four miles, thanks to my vascular surgeon. My team got off together but we became separated because there were so many walkers. My husband had to do the shorter route, but he was there for me, bad knees and all. Other team members also chose the two-mile route for various reasons, but my vascular surgeon gave me the legs to walk for anyone who couldn't. I finished the last two miles by myself. I smiled the entire way. I didn't feel alone. I felt empowered. I cried!

I will walk every year, even if it is by myself. This walk did give me a new strength. I expect it will give me strength every single year.

REMEMBER, ANYONE CAN LOVE YOU WHEN THE SUN IS SHINING... IT'S DURING THE STORMS WHEN YOU FIND OUT WHO REALLY CARES!

I see things a lot differently now.

To quote a line from a favorite movie, *Last Holiday*, "Time is rather precious these days." To realize your own mortality is humbling. To understand who is willing to take this walk with you is eye-opening. You just never know what is waiting around the next corner for you. Time IS precious.

We prepare for everything throughout our lives. We study for tests. We take classes to prepare for SATs. We pay fees on sites to help us write the perfect resume for that gotta-have job. We role-play for job interviews. We even buy and read books about planning weddings and bringing up babies. Why would you not prepare yourself for how to support your wife, mother, best friend, or sister?

Everyone knows or will know someone affected by a potentially life-changing diagnosis. Why would you not prepare yourself for a life-changing experience and be a better person for it? Why? It won't happen to you?

Think again!

One out of eight women in the United States will be diagnosed with breast cancer in their lifetime. There was no history of breast cancer in my family. I do not carry any of the genes known to cause breast cancer, yet, I was last year's 1 out of 8—that is a 12.5% risk!

What are your chances of winning the lottery? A quick look at the lottery website tells you the probability of winning the Powerball jackpot is approximately 1 in 175,223,510. Yet people play and play and play.

Be prepared!

Know what to say, or, more important, what NOT to say! Think about what you can do to brighten someone's day or how you could make a difference for them.

If only one person now understands the risk to them or a sister, mother, or daughter, then I will consider this story to have been successful. I want EVERYONE to hear, loud and clear, this message long before they or their wife, mother, sister, or friend hears, "We think we saw something on your mammogram."

There is a laundry list of things that can contribute to cancer, but I know there are thousands of women out there, just like me, who never once gave breast cancer a thought let alone a worry because it didn't run in their family. It doesn't have to run in your family.

The sister of my cousin who had the breast cancer, while taking hormone replacements, would also be diagnosed with breast cancer a few months after me. All three of us were genetically tested. None of us carries the BRCA genes. Our genetics panels were clear. We have not lived in the same states since college, which is more than 30 years ago. We were just part of that 1 out of 8. Interesting, isn't it?

I hope my story makes women aware that the number-one risk to breast cancer is being a woman.

I discovered throughout my research that only 65%–70% of U.S. women get a yearly mammogram (Mammography, 2016). My walk was not easy, but it was much easier and shorter than so many others. Small stints of short-term radiation for a yearly mammogram is far less intrusive than 40 full-dose radiation treatments for cancer, not to mention the possibility of the chemotherapy drugs. And once a year doesn't take up nearly as much time as those 40 trips to the hospital every single day! Knowledge truly is power!

I write my story to make everyone aware that there is nothing simple about any of this. It is endless appointments with surgeons, radiation oncologists, radiologists, medical oncologists, technicians, immunotherapists, and possibly plastic surgeons. There are endless side effects to everything. You, my family and friends never see the warnings in the endless release forms that we are required to sign. No one ever asks you, "Would you prefer this side effect or that?" I suppose we keep it to ourselves so you don't worry. This can be life-changing and overwhelming, not just physically but mentally. None of it is easy, no matter what anyone tells you.

I write my story to shout from the rooftop, "It's ok to resent the hand you have been dealt. It is just a lousy hand no matter how you look at it. Don't let anyone tell you it's not!" You are not alone in these feelings. It's ok to have those feelings!

I had a newly diagnosed cancer patient ask me to explain what "plan" I had been given. When I explained my treatment regimen she responded, "I don't have time for that! I have a benefit to plan and a party I'm hosting and we have planned our yearly family vacation." None of us has time for any of this, but what choice is there? Please don't look down on us because we found this challenge to be just a bit too much. Support us, somehow.

I write my story to say that words have meaning. Words also have consequences.

Sometimes you just need a hug; no words needed!

Please make time in your busy life for those you love.

Think before you speak! Please choose your words very carefully. This could be you next year. Would you want to be told not to worry, only to be diagnosed with cancer and spend the next year and possibly more going through chemotherapy and radiation? How neatly does that fit into your world?

My friend who has the cousin with breast cancer came to me the other day and showed me a picture of his cousin where she had shaved her head. She was about to begin her chemotherapy treatments. He asked me why she did that. I told him maybe she feels more in control. Maybe it is easier for her to look in the mirror at what she did to herself, rather than to have a handful of red curls in her hand in the shower tomorrow from what the treatments did to her today.

I've walked past a lot of chemotherapy rooms and hoped they could feel me sending strength. I don't know how they do it. What's the alternative? What other choice is there? We are fortunate to have the medical technology.

It's unfortunate how it can forever affect and change your life and be so very cruel. I hope my experience helps to improve the twists and turns we are expected to endure. Maybe that hallway door will finally have an automated closure installed, please!

I've sat in a lot of cancer patient waiting rooms and have observed young mothers with children. How do they do it? I've seen the sickness in so many of their eyes. How do they get through? I hope they have lots of shoulders to lean on and arms to hug them. I hope no one is told, "Don't worry, it won't be cancer" or told how lucky they are since so much is known about breast cancer. Yes, these are statements that people I know have heard from friends and family.

I suppose I could have handled things better, but 36 days of not knowing what the future held for me was just too much. I just couldn't handle one more, "We saved your leg" or "Next time we may have to amputate your finger." I had 36 days and 36 nights to hear those words run through my mind again and again. I guess I had hoped my family and friends would have remembered all that I had been through and understood why I was so distressed.

My vascular surgeon told me, "You will get through with your great resolve." We all get through it, but there are a lot of bumps and bruises along the way. He was right. I got through it, but not very gracefully.

I'm telling my story not because my cancer diagnosis was unique, but to point out how even the most positive prognosis with what most would consider a simple treatment plan will consume your life. People's actions or, more importantly, inactions can forever change you as a person. Make time in your life. Don't let anyone ever feel alone and abandoned when they are up against any medical diagnosis. My hope is that at least one new person will understand how to support their wife, daughter, sister, or friend. Even the most graceful people I know with words didn't know what to do for or say to me, and truly stepped right in it and made things worse.

No one is likely to run out and buy a book once they are diagnosed with cancer or any other disease. They are going to stare at their doctor or nurse, nod their heads, and walk away with an armful of brochures and pamphlets about ductal carcinoma, invasive versus noninvasive, edema therapy, hormone receptors, or lymphedema. All words that you will likely later have to look up. After a few months of all of this, you could pass a medical terminology class with an "A."

So, prepare how to handle the moment.

This could be you, your wife, a friend, or even your daughter. At any given moment, this shoe could be on your foot.

IF I KNEW THEN, WHAT I KNOW NOW...
BUT I WANT YOU TO KNOW!

I would end up taking a few classes at the community college. I was required to do a medical research paper. I chose Breast Cancer. What I learned had my head spinning.

Here are a few of those head-spinning statistics regarding breast cancer.

Approximately 1 out of 8 U.S. women (about 12.5%) will develop invasive breast cancer in their lifetime (Breastcancer.org, 2017). It was also estimated that in 2017 approximately 40,610 American women would die from breast cancer (Breast Cancer, 2017).

The Susan G. Komen foundation estimated that in 2017 there would be 252,710 new cases of invasive breast cancer among women in the United States (Breast Cancer, 2017). The Susan G. Komen foundation anticipated that in 2016 there would be some "246,600 new cases of invasive breast cancer. (This includes new cases of primary breast cancer among survivors.)" (Breast Cancer, 2016). That is an increase from one year to the next by more than a 2%. They also anticipated "61,000 new cases of in situ breast cancer. (This includes ductal carcinoma in situ (DCIS) and lobular carcinoma in situ (LCIS).)" (komen.org, 2016).

A woman's risk of breast cancer nearly doubles if she has a first-degree relative (mother, sister, daughter) who has been diagnosed with breast cancer. Less than 15% of women who get breast cancer have a family member diagnosed with it. For women in the United States, breast cancer death rates are higher than those for any other cancer, besides lung cancer (Breastcancer.org, 2017).

Approximately 85% of breast cancer occurs in women with no family history of breast cancer. This occurs due to a genetic mutation that can occur as a result of the aging process rather than inherited mutations (Breastcancer.org, 2017).

Many factors known to increase the risk of breast cancer are not modifiable, such as age, family history, early menarche, and late menopause (American Cancer Society, 2015–2016, p. 11).

Other factors that increase the risk for cancer are as follows:

- Alcohol consumption
- Diet
- Exercise
- High estrogen levels
- Hormone use
- Late age for first full-term pregnancy
- Never breast-feeding
- Not having children
- Recent, oral contraceptive use
- Stress
- Tobacco use
- Weight gain

According to the CDC's most recent statistics, each year approximately 68% of American women go for a yearly mammography screening (cdc.gov, 2016). That means that approximately 32% do not.

Cancer is defined as "uncontrolled growth of cells in the human body and the ability of these cells to migrate from the original site and spread to distant sites" (*Mosby's*, 2013), or to metastasize.

The two most significant risk factors for breast cancer are age and being a woman (Breastcancer.org, 2017).

"As of March 2017, there are more than 3.1 million women with a history of breast cancer in the U.S. This includes women being treated and women who have finished treatment" (Breastcancer. org, 2017).

"Besides skin cancer, breast cancer is the most commonly diagnosed cancer among American women. In 2017, it's estimated that just below 30% of newly diagnosed cancers in women will be breast cancer" (Breastcancer.org, 2017).

So why didn't I know that breast cancer is the second-leading cause of death of U.S. women? According to the American Heart Association, "while 1 in 31 American women dies from breast cancer each year, 1 in 3 dies of heart disease" (heart.org, 2017).

Cancer is the second most common cause of death in the United States, second only to heart disease (heart.org, 2017).

Although rare, pre-menopausal women also get breast cancer. Fewer than 5% of the cases occur in women under the age of 40 yet breast cancer is the leading cause of cancer death (death from any type of cancer) among women ages 20-39 (komen.org, 2017).

While the next part is merely my speculation, it is based on much research. According to my research, the female body is producing too much estrogen and the following are possible signals or signs that this occurring. I had every one of these signals as I entered menopause.

1. Heavy and Irregular Menstrual Cycles
2. Swelling or changes in breast size
3. Hypothyroidism
4. Decrease Sex Drive
5. Mood Swings
6. Cold Hands & Feet
7. High Blood Pressure

8.   Uterine Fibroids
9.   Acne

This site has a good explanation for this...
http://www.healthyyounaturally.com/edu/women-dangers.htm
When I asked my gynecologist about the breast changes, she shrugged it off to fatty tissue deposits. I asked her if I looked fat?
I wished I had known.

IT'S BEEN A VERY LONG YEAR

It is now December 16th. It's approaching the one-year mark when I was completely blindsided by "12.5 % of U.S. women will be diagnosed this year with breast cancer, while some 40,000 plus will die from it" (Breastcancer.org, 2017). And that has nothing to do with genetics.

I'm waiting for my first mammogram since my cancer diagnosis. I am not looking forward to that machine compressing my breast. Believe it or not, it is still slightly sore and slightly swollen. My breast just isn't the same. It is hard and dense. That will most definitely resist the compression. Sometimes at the end of the day, it feels like little pins and needles on my skin as my bra moves against it. It's been nearly six months since my last radiation treatment. I'm told by a friend, six years post cancer, that this is the way it will be. I guess this is what you would call a long-term side effect. This is my new normal.

As I'm waiting, I meet a woman a bit younger than me. She is telling me she makes a two-hour drive once a week to come to this well-known cancer center for her chemotherapy. Her tumor was so large and aggressive they could not operate. She will be doing this for weeks, if not months, to help shrink it, and then they will operate. Then there may be more chemotherapy, then on to 6 or more weeks of radiation and potentially another round of chemotherapy.

She confides in me that she just wants her life back. She tells me she is doing better than when she was first diagnosed and that she is "trying to be happy." Her husband doesn't understand, but she really is "trying to be happy." I know it's hard. I understand. There is nothing easy about any of this.

If you are reading this, I hope it helps you understand. This disrupts your life. It disrupts your world. It doesn't just affect you physically. It beats you up mentally. I wonder if anyone told her not to worry?

She is wearing a wig, God bless her. Neither of us has the genetic markers. We are just part of that 1 out of 8.

I would have my mammogram and be given the all clear, for now. My eyes were full of tears. I asked my technician if I could hug her. I texted my husband from the changing room with the news. I didn't want to skip into the larger waiting room grinning from ear to ear. Many out there are not getting good news today.

Year one down, many more to go. The first three years are the most crucial, my oncologist tells me. Cancer may never be part of my life again, but it could be at any moment for me or for anyone. Age is up there on the risk factor list and NONE of us are getting any younger.

Later, my surgeon would hug me and say, "You are all my heroes." I don't feel like a hero. I was scared. I still am. I suppose time will help heal and give me more strength. I hope!

I just want all the friends and family members out there to realize this isn't just a blip on a screen. It's cancer. It's not a skinned knee. It isn't just one surgery or a few trips to the local hospital. It is life changing. Cancer patients will forever be looking over their shoulders. There is no cure.

How to begin, how to deal with it, and how to make a plan to move forward can be overwhelming (Brokaw, 2014) without a roadmap of what to expect.

I know there is someone out there reading this saying that they wished that they had my simpler treatment schedule. Yes, in hindsight my walk was simpler than so many others. I know that there are some very long and complicated cancer walks out there. I wish no one had to endure any of this, but I write my story so that maybe just one person will do things differently and make a cancer patient's life just a little easier, or their day a little brighter.

So, choose your words carefully. It isn't over quickly. It isn't a piece of cake. We have every right to be worried. We have every right to be mad and angry. We have every right to act like three-year-old's. It's ok to ask, "why me?" Nothing is easy about any of this. And it never goes away.

Don't be silent. Offer support somehow. One former coworker just hugged me when I told her. Nothing else was said. Show your support with a text, greeting card, telephone call, email, flowers, baked cookies, invitation for coffee or lunch, offer of a ride, a surprise visit, post a cheer on their website, or just give them a simple hug. Understand that this goes on and on. Continue to show your support. Don't let any cancer patient feel alone or forgotten. They may have won this battle but the war is by no means over.

Make time in your busy day.

Try to walk in their shoes for just a moment.

And hope that you are not next year's 12.5%.

Ask them how they are doing. They will thank you for asking.

MY RULES OF THE ROAD

It doesn't matter what challenge your "best buddie" is facing, the rules of the road are the same. Be there, in some way shape or form, but be there! Support your "friend."

1. Send flowers! This is non-negotiable!
2. Send well wishes in the form of greeting cards, emails or text message. Set a reminder on YOUR phone to do it often. Also, non-negotiable!!
3. Listen! You don't need to offer advice or try to come up with some cliché' about how cancer is a journey and she'll get through it because she's strong. **Just listen!**
4. Accept their coping mechanism. Everyone handles stress differently. They have to endure and live through it, you don't!
5. Make their day a little easier and gift a housekeeper, manicure, dinner delivered or some fun treat! Make them smile!
6. Offer your ears, arms, shoulders and TIME. Don't be too busy. Don't disappear when the going gets tough. Make a special trip to be with them.
7. Focus on the person, not the illness & DO NOT COMPARE PEOPLE!

8. Tell her you're there for her, and mean it. Ask what you can do. Ask how you can help. Be sincere. Make time and give time.
9. Do not offer medical advice!
10. Just because it's been a few months since a diagnosis, do it all over again & again & again!

Since my breast cancer experience, I think I'm single-handedly giving new life to the greeting card industry. I buy and send them often these days. It meant the world to me to receive one.

Now with my top 10-list in hand, you can truly support your friend, sister, mother or daughter. Well, at least it's a start!

Brighten someone's day with a kind gesture. You have no idea how much something as simple as a 99-cent greeting card could mean.

Keep this top ten list handy, always!

EPILOGUE

Two years have passed since that dust-bunny was seen on my mammogram. I'd be lying if I didn't tell you that I worry each day about the cancer returning; it does for way too many. I will always be looking over my shoulder, but we all should. I'm learning to live with my fears. But I finally now know that I'm not alone; I'm not alone in my fears, frustrations and crazy experiences. I now know that I'm not crazy or broken because of my worries. It would be utterly unrealistic to expect someone to be fearless when faced with cancer.

Time does help. Time does help heal.

My year taught me many valuable lessons. It showed me the real meaning of friendship and the true meaning of support. Because of that, I think my husband and I are better people for those facing medical challenges or any challenge for that matter. He too discovered that words have meaning and things are not always what they seem. He now knows that a cancer diagnosis is life-changing. He is anxiously awaiting the release of my book, to know how best to be there for his co-worker.

We both have co-workers with challenging cancer diagnoses. We take the time to check in with them, send cards, send flowers and ask what we can do. We are practicing what I have been preaching and the two of us may just give new life to the greeting card industry.

I heard at a seminar, "everyone has a story to tell." That is why I kept on writing.

What made me finally decide to publish my thoughts, fears, emotions, and crazy experiences was that I think I might be making a difference after all.

I had breakfast with an old friend not long ago and told her about my long, long year. She telephoned the other day, and during the conversation, she stated, "I was going to forgo my mammogram this year, but after what you told me, I'm not."

Then my sister-in-law confided after reading my blog, "OK, overdue . . . calling to make appointments first thing Monday."

I was speaking with a young woman the other day who just unexpectedly lost a family member at the age of 28. She told me she had been avoiding his parents because she didn't know what to say. I suggested that she just give them a hug and that no words were needed. She turned and a big smile came over her face. She said, "You're right!"

Maybe I can shout from the rooftops and make a difference after all. Maybe you will take the time to buy that greeting card or send that text and brighten someone's else's day. Maybe my facility will fix that door with an automated closing device and give someone else just a bit more dignity. Maybe there will finally be a commercial that states, "It's ok to be worried and afraid." Maybe someone will update those handouts at the treatment centers and "hugging can be hazardous" will finally be listed. Maybe our friends and family will bite their tongue and not say, "You are strong and I know you can get through this."

Or maybe, just maybe our friends and family will just hug us and ask how they can help.

I can hope.

I hope my story makes a difference for you.

I hope it makes a difference for someone you love.

FOLLOW MY BLOG AT

https://nogenesneeded.com/

Please join me and tell your experiences; the good, the bad & the ugly. Let other woman know they are not alone with their feelings, fears, emotions and crazy experiences.

Maybe together we can all make a difference and make one person's experience just a little easier.

SEND FLOWERS, OFTEN! – August 28, 2017
It doesn't matter what challenge your "best buddie" is facing, the rules of the road are the same. Be there, in some way shape or form, but be there! Support your "friend."

WHAT ARE THE CHANCES? – September 13, 2017
Why do we wait until October to talk about Breast Cancer? If no one is going print these statistics year-round, then ladies we need to talk about it and spread the word!

It's 1 out of 8, no genes required!

THE BIG UGLY MACHINE – September 24, 2017
There are certain yearly appointments that you never look forward to; the dentist, the gynecologist and the mammogram. I don't know why exactly, as much as they are just unpleasant and awkward.

MY BEST FRIEND – October 18, 2017

We all have a best friend in our lives. Some we have known since Kindergarten. Others you met in college or at work. Some of our best friends, we married. And yet others we have known our entire lives and call them brother or sister.

HERE'S YOUR SIGN – October 29, 2017

But why is it when you are potentially facing bad news the strangest and sometimes hurtful things come out of the mouths of people you love?

Some friends and family become a bunch of cheerleaders with, "think positive thoughts," or "you must believe your glass is half full" or "it won't happen to you."

THE NEW NORMAL – November 11, 2017

I re-read those endless brochures and pamphlets that I had been given in the beginning. Yes, they mention *slight swelling* and firmness but I wished they had listed, "Caution during hugs!".

MONDAY MORNING QUARTERBACKING – December 22, 2017

It's quite easy to tell someone else what they should do or how they should do it when they have never faced it themselves.

Monday morning quarterbacking….as they say!

WHAT WILL YOU DO WHEN SHE'S NOT THERE – December 31, 2017

My sister needed me. She needed my advice on her daughter's fever. She had a sister to call.

Don't wait for tomorrow, live today!

REFERENCES

American Cancer Society. *Breast Cancer Facts & Figures 2015–2016*. Web. June 20, 2016. www.cancer.org/acs/groups/content/@ research/documents/document/acspc-046381.pdf.

Breast Cancer Global Statistics at Susan G. Komen. May 17, 2016. komen.org. Retrieved June 4, 2016. ww5.komen.org/ BreastCancer/Statistics.html.

Breast Cancer Global Statistics at Susan G. Komen. June 5, 2017. komen.org. Retrieved August 1, 2017. ww5.komen.org/ BreastCancer/Statistics.html.

Brokaw, T. (November 19, 2014) Join Visiting Committee Dinner [Video file]. Retrieved 19 June 2016. https://www.youtube.com/ watch?v=0uudn6JlAxo

The Heart Foundation. www.theheartfoundation.org/heart-disease-facts/heart-disease-statistics/ Retrieved August 1, 2017

Centers for Disease Control and Prevention. "Mammography and Breast Cancer." April 27, 2016. Web. June 21, 2016. www.cdc. gov/nchs/fastats/mammography.htm.

Mosby's Dictionary of Medicine, Nursing & Health Professions. 9th ed. St. Louis, MO: Elsevier/Mosby, 2013. Print.

Treatment for DCIS at Susan G. Komen. Recommended Treatments for Ductal Carcinoma in Situ. March 18, 2016. Retrieved June 4, 2016. ww5.komen.org/BreastCancer/ RecommendedTreatmentsforDuctalCarcinomaInSitu.html.

"U.S. Breast Cancer Statistics." Breastcancer.org. N.p., March 10, 2017. Web. August 1, 2017. www.breastcancer.org/symptoms/ understand_bc/statistics.

U.S. Food and Drug Administration. fda.gov.